THE COMPLETE PEGAN DIET COOKBOOK

COMBINE THE BEST OF PALEO AND VEGAN DIET FOR LIFELONG HEALTH.

The Healthier Press

TABLE OF CONTENTS:

CHAPTER 1: BREAKFAST RECIPES 6

   EGG AND AVOCADO TOAST 7
   STRAWBERRY BANANA PROTEIN SMOOTHIE 9
   TOMATO, FENNEL AND WATERCRESS SALAD 11
   AVOCADO CHICKEN LETTUCE WRAPS 13
   CREPES WITH SPINACH, BACON AND MUSHROOM FILLING 15
   PALEO BAKED EGGS IN AVOCADO 18
   CREAMY COTTAGE CHEESE SCRAMBLED EGGS 20
   CAULIFLOWER AND SWEET POTATO HASH 22
   SPICY POTATOES AND SCRAMBLED EGGS 24
   CINNAMON APPLES 26
   GREEN EGGS AND HASH OMELET 27
   BAKED DEVILED EGGS WITH ASPARAGUS 29
   SPICY SWEET PEPPER POPPERS 32

CHAPTER 2: LUNCH RECIPES 35

   TURKEY VEGGIE MEATLOAF CUPS 36
   ONION AND MUSHROOM SCRAMBLED EGGS 38
   CREAMY, LEMONY POTATO SALAD 40
   SPICY SWEET POTATO AND COCONUT SOUP 42
   POTATO-FREE PALEO GNOCCHI 44
   CUCUMBER WATERMELON SALAD 46
   MUSHROOM, SCALLION, AND CHEESE OMELET 48
   PRETZEL TOPPED SWEET POTATOES 50
   SAUTEED RICE WITH KALE 52
   TENDER ONION BAKED CHICKEN 54
   MAYO FREE CABBAGE SALAD 56
   SWEET AND TANGY APPLE PORK CHOPS 58
   CURRIED MUSTARD GREENS WITH KIDNEY BEANS 60
   CREAMED BROCCOLI SOUP 62

CHAPTER 3: DINNER RECIPES 65

   SPICY SALMON AND VEGETABLE BOWL 66
   HOMEMADE VEGETABLE BEEF SOUP 69
   LEMONY SALMON WITH WATERCRESS SALAD 71

CARROT, TOMATO, AND SPINACH QUINOA PILAF WITH GROUND TURKEY 74
SAVORY VEGETABLE BEEF STEW 77
AMAZING GRILLED CHICKEN AND PINEAPPLE 79
FRESH VEGETABLE STIR-FRY WITH PEPPERY ORANGE BEEF...................... 82
BACON ROSEMARY STUFFED MUSHROOMS 85
CLASSIC BEEF STUFFED PEPPERS.. 87
CRANBERRY AND TURKEY SALAD... 89
TURKEY VEGETABLE SOUP 90
PEANUT BUTTER SAUCE CHICKEN.. 92
ASIAGO TOASTED CHEESE PUFFS 94
SPICY ORANGE CHICKEN 96

CHAPTER 4: SMOOTHIE RECIPES 100
BANANA-DATE SHAKE 101
SWEET POTATO-BANANA SMOOTHIE 102
STRAWBERRY-ORANGE CREME SMOOTHIES... 104
VANILLA BANAMANGO SMOOTHIE 106
ZUCCHINI SMOOTHIE... 108

© Copyright 2021 by The Healthier Press All rights reserved.

The following Book is reproduced below with the goal of providing information that is as accurate and reliable as possible. Regardless, purchasing this Book can be seen as consent to the fact that both the publisher and the author of this book are in no way experts on the topics discussed within and that any recommendations or suggestions that are made herein are for entertainment purposes only. Professionals should be consulted as needed prior to undertaking any of the action endorsed herein.

This declaration is deemed fair and valid by both the American Bar Association and the Committee of Publishers Association and is legally binding throughout the United States.

Furthermore, the transmission, duplication, or reproduction of any of the following work including specific information will be considered an illegal act irrespective of if it is done electronically or in print. This extends to creating a secondary or tertiary copy of the work or a recorded copy and is only allowed with the express written consent from the Publisher. All additional right reserved.

The information in the following pages is broadly considered a truthful and accurate account of facts and as such, any inattention, use, or misuse of the information in question by the reader will render any resulting actions solely under their purview. There are no scenarios in which the publisher or the original author of this work can be in any fashion deemed liable for any hardship or damages that may befall them after undertaking information described herein.

Additionally, the information in the following pages is intended only for informational purposes and should thus be thought of as universal. As befitting its nature, it is presented without assurance regarding its prolonged validity or interim quality. Trademarks that are mentioned are done without written consent and can in no way be considered an endorsement from the trademark holder.

CHAPTER 1: BREAKFAST RECIPES

EGG AND AVOCADO TOAST

Prep:
5 mins
Cook:
5 mins
Total:
10 mins
Servings:
1
Yield:
1 avocado toast

INGREDIENTS:

1 slice multigrain seeded sandwich bread
½ teaspoon vegetable oil
1 egg
flaky sea salt to taste
freshly ground black pepper to taste
2 pinches red pepper flakes
½ ripe avocado
1 wedge lemon

DIRECTIONS:

Step 1
Toast bread on the highest setting until dark golden brown all over.

Step 2
Heat a small pan over medium heat. Brush oil onto the hot pan and crack in the egg. Sprinkle sea salt, black pepper, and pepper flakes on top. Cover and cook until whites are set and yolk is still runny, about 3 minutes.

Step 3
Scoop avocado onto the toast and spread evenly.
 Squeeze some lemon juice on top.
Season with salt, black pepper, and red pepper flakes.
Top with fried egg; pierce the yolk
and spread it around.
Squeeze in more lemon juice to taste and cut avocado toast in half for optimal enjoyment.

NUTRITION FACTS:

333 calories; protein 12.3g; carbohydrates 23.5g; fat 23.5g; cholesterol 186mg; sodium 507.7mg.

STRAWBERRY BANANA PROTEIN SMOOTHIE

Prep:
10 mins
Total:
10 mins
Servings:
1
Yield:
1 smoothie

INGREDIENTS:

1 banana
1 ¼ cups sliced fresh strawberries
10 whole almonds
2 tablespoons water
1 cup ice cubes
3 tablespoons chocolate flavored protein powder

DIRECTIONS:

Step 1
Place the banana, strawberries, almonds, and water into a blender. Blend to mix, then add the ice cubes and puree until smooth. Add the protein powder, and continue mixing until evenly incorporated, about 30 seconds.

NUTRITION FACTS:

349 calories; protein 21g; carbohydrates 53.2g; fat 8.1g; sodium 194.5mg

TOMATO, FENNEL AND WATERCRESS SALAD

Prep:
15 mins
Total:
15 mins
Servings:
6
Yield:
6 servings

INGREDIENTS:

2 tablespoons white wine vinegar
4 teaspoons chopped fresh tarragon
2 teaspoons Dijon-style prepared mustard
1 teaspoon fennel seed, ground
5 tablespoons olive oil
3 cups trimmed and coarsely chopped watercress
2 bulbs fennel, trimmed and thinly sliced
6 large tomatoes

DIRECTIONS:

Step 1
Whisk together the vinegar, tarragon, mustard, fennel seed and olive oil.

Step 2
Cut the tomatoes into 1/2 inch thick wedges. In a large salad bowl, combine the watercress, fennel and tomatoes. Toss with vinaigrette to coat, season with salt and pepper and serve.

NUTRITION FACTS:

162 calories; protein 3.1g; carbohydrates 13.6g; fat 11.9g;

AVOCADO CHICKEN LETTUCE WRAPS

Prep:
10 mins
Cook:
40 mins
Additional:
10 mins
Total:
1 hr
Servings:
4
Yield:
4 servings

INGREDIENTS:

2 boneless, skinless chicken breasts
2 tablespoons olive oil
2 teaspoons mango lime seasoning blend
1 large avocado - peeled, pitted, and diced
2 tablespoons lime juice, or more to taste
2 tablespoons hot salsa (Optional)
1 tablespoon chopped fresh cilantro, or more to taste
1 tablespoon garlic powder
salt and ground black pepper to taste
1 head romaine lettuce, leaves separated

DIRECTIONS:

Step 1
Preheat oven to 300 degrees F (150 degrees C).

Step 2
Coat chicken breasts with olive oil and sprinkle mango and lime seasoning on both sides. Place in a shallow baking dish and cover with aluminum foil.

Step 3
Bake chicken in the preheated oven until no longer pink in the center and an instant-read thermometer inserted into the center reads at least 165 degrees F (74 degrees C), 40 to 45 minutes. Remove from oven and cool until easily handled, about 10 minutes.

Step 4
Chop chicken into small pieces and place in a large bowl. Add avocado, lime juice, salsa, cilantro, garlic powder, salt, and black pepper; mix well to combine. Serve on top of lettuce leaves to make wraps.

NUTRITION FACTS:

264 calories; protein 15.2g; carbohydrates 11.5g; fat 18.9g; cholesterol 33.6mg;

CREPES WITH SPINACH, BACON AND MUSHROOM FILLING

Prep:
35 mins
Cook:
20 mins
Total:
1 hr 5 mins

INGREDIENTS:

1 recipe Basic Crepes
6 slices bacon
1 tablespoon unsalted butter
½ pound fresh mushrooms, sliced
3 tablespoons unsalted butter
¼ cup all-purpose flour
1 cup milk
1 (10 ounce) package frozen chopped spinach, thawed and drained
1 tablespoon chopped fresh parsley
2 tablespoons grated Parmesan cheese
salt and pepper to taste
⅔ cup chicken broth
2 eggs
½ cup lemon juice
salt and pepper to taste

DIRECTIONS:

Step 1
Prepare Basic Crepes recipe according to recipe directions. Separate with wax paper and keep warm until ready to serve.

Step 2
Place bacon in a large, deep skillet. Cook over medium-high heat until evenly brown. Drain, crumble and set aside. Reserve about 1 tablespoon drippings, add 1 tablespoon butter, and saute mushrooms.

Step 3
In a separate saucepan, melt 3 tablespoons butter over medium heat. Whisk in 1/4 cup flour, stirring constantly, until a smooth paste is formed. Gradually stir in 1 cup milk, stirring constantly until a smooth thick gravy is formed. Add bacon, mushrooms, spinach, parsley, Parmesan cheese, salt and pepper. Let cook until somewhat thick, about 10 minutes.

Step 4
In saucepan bring broth to a boil. In a small bowl, whisk together eggs and lemon juice. Temper eggs and broth together whisking constantly so as to cook, but not to scramble the eggs. (Cooking eggs to 170 degrees F). Again, salt and pepper to taste.

Step 5
Fill each crepe with spinach and meat filling, roll up, and top with warm egg sauce.

NUTRITION FACTS:

445 calories; protein 15.9g; carbohydrates 17.9g; fat 35.6g; cholesterol 160mg;

PALEO BAKED EGGS IN AVOCADO

Prep:
10 mins
Cook:
15 mins
Total:
25 mins
Servings:
2
Yield:
2 servings

INGREDIENTS:

2 small eggs
1 avocado, halved and pitted
2 slices cooked bacon, crumbled
2 teaspoons chopped fresh chives, or to taste
1 pinch dried parsley, or to taste
1 pinch sea salt and ground black pepper to taste

18

DIRECTIONS:

Instructions Checklist
Step 1
Preheat oven to 425 degrees F (220 degrees C).

Step 2
Crack the eggs into a bowl, being careful to keep the yolks intact.

Step 3
Arrange avocado halves in a baking dish, resting them along the edge so avocado won't tip over. Gently spoon 1 egg yolk into the avocado hole. Continue spooning egg white into the hole until full. Repeat with remaining egg yolk, egg white, and avocado. Season each filled avocado with chives, parsley, sea salt, and pepper.

Step 4
Gently place baking dish in the preheated oven and bake until eggs are cooked, about 15 minutes. Sprinkle bacon over avocado.

NUTRITION FACTS:

280 calories; protein 11.3g; carbohydrates 9.3g; fat 23.5g; cholesterol 150.8mg

CREAMY COTTAGE CHEESE SCRAMBLED EGGS

Prep:
5 mins
Cook:
5 mins
Total:
10 mins
Servings:
2
Yield:
2 servings

INGREDIENTS:

1 tablespoon butter
4 eggs, beaten
¼ cup cottage cheese
ground black pepper to taste
1 teaspoon chopped fresh chives, or to taste (Optional)

DIRECTIONS:

Step 1
Melt butter in a skillet over medium heat. Pour beaten eggs into the skillet; let cook undisturbed until the bottom of the eggs begin to firm, 1 to 2 minutes.

Step 2
Stir cottage cheese and chives into eggs and season with black pepper. Cook and stir until eggs are nearly set, 3 to 4 minutes more.

NUTRITION FACTS:

224 calories; protein 16.2g; carbohydrates 1.9g; fat 17g; cholesterol 391.5mg;

CAULIFLOWER AND SWEET POTATO HASH

Prep:
15 mins
Cook:
9 mins
Total:
24 mins
Servings:
4
Yield:
4 servings

INGREDIENTS:

2 tablespoons olive oil
1 small onion, chopped
1 (12 ounce) package Green Giant® Riced Cauliflower & Sweet Potato
1 red bell pepper, chopped
2 cloves garlic, minced
½ teaspoon salt
2 cups fresh baby kale or spinach
1 teaspoon sriracha hot chile sauce, or to taste
4 large eggs eggs, fried or poached

DIRECTIONS:

Step 1
Heat olive oil in large nonstick skillet over medium-high heat and cook onion 3 minutes or until softened.

Step 2
Stir in Green Giant® Riced Cauliflower and Sweet Potatoes, red pepper, garlic and salt and cook 5 minutes, stirring occasionally, or until vegetables are tender.

Step 3
Stir in kale and cook 2 minutes or until wilted. Stir in sriracha.

Step 4
Serve eggs over hash

NUTRITION FACTS:

236 calories; protein 10g; carbohydrates 18.8g; fat 14.1g; cholesterol 184.5mg; sodium 474.3mg.

SPICY POTATOES AND SCRAMBLED EGGS

Prep:
10 mins
Cook:
15 mins
Total:
25 mins
Servings:
4
Yield:
3 to 4 servings

INGREDIENTS:

2 potatoes, scrubbed
4 tablespoons vegetable oil, divided
3 eggs
salt and pepper to taste
½ teaspoon ground cumin
½ teaspoon ground coriander
½ teaspoon turmeric powder
½ teaspoon chili powder
½ teaspoon salt

DIRECTIONS:

Step 1

Poke potatoes with a fork so that their skins are pierced. Microwave potatoes on high until cooked inside. When potatoes are fully cooked, peel potatoes and cut potatoes to 1/8 size or to your liking. Set potatoes aside.

Step 2

Add 2 tablespoons oil to skillet and scramble 3 eggs. Add salt and pepper to taste. Keep warm until potatoes are ready.

Step 3

In another skillet, heat 2 tablespoons oil until hot.
Then add salt, cumin, coriander
and turmeric powder.
Put in chili powder if you want it really spicy.
Add potatoes and cook
until potatoes are crispy and brown.
Spicy potatoes and scrambled
eggs are now ready to serve!

NUTRITION FACTS:

209 calories; protein 5.5g; carbohydrates 8.2g; fat 17.5g; cholesterol 139.5mg;

CINNAMON APPLES

Prep:
5 mins
Cook:
2 mins
Total:
7 mins
Servings:
4
Yield:
4 servings

INGREDIENTS:

2 apples, diced
1 teaspoon white sugar
½ teaspoon ground cinnamon

DIRECTIONS:

Step 1
Place apples in a microwave-safe bowl; heat in microwave for 30 seconds. Sprinkle sugar and cinnamon over apples and stir to coat. Heat apples in microwave until soft and warm, about 1 minute more.

NUTRITION FACTS:

41 calories; protein 0.2g; carbohydrates 10.8g; fat 0.1g; sodium 0.7mg.

GREEN EGGS AND HASH OMELET

Prep:
10 mins
Cook:
6 mins
Total:
16 mins
Servings:
1
Yield:
1 omelet

INGREDIENTS:

2 eggs
2 cups loosely packed fresh spinach
1 cup corned beef hash
freshly ground black pepper to taste
cooking spray
2 tablespoons shredded mozzarella cheese, or to taste

DIRECTIONS:

Step 1
Combine eggs and spinach in a blender. Blend on high speed for 1 minute. Scrape down the sides of the blender. Pulse until spinach is fully blended into the eggs, about 1 minute more.

Step 2
Pour hash into a microwave-safe bowl. Heat in the microwave until thoroughly warmed, about 1 minute. Season with black pepper.

Step 3
Spray a nonstick skillet with cooking spray; place over medium heat.
Pour in egg-spinach mixture. Cover with a lid.
Cook until top is barely set, about 5 minutes.
Place corned beef hash over 1 side of the omelet.
Slide onto a plate,
using the skillet to fold the other side on top.
Sprinkle mozzarella cheese over omelet.

NUTRITION FACTS:

596 calories; protein 37.2g; carbohydrates 27.5g; fat 37.6g; cholesterol 453.6mg;

BAKED DEVILED EGGS WITH ASPARAGUS

Prep:
30 mins
Cook:
30 mins
Total:
1 hr

INGREDIENTS:

2 pounds fresh asparagus, trimmed and cut into 1-inch pieces
10 hard-cooked eggs, peeled and sliced in half lengthwise
1 (4.5 ounce) can deviled ham spread
1 tablespoon heavy cream
1 teaspoon grated onion
¾ teaspoon dry mustard powder
½ teaspoon Worcestershire sauce
½ teaspoon salt
6 tablespoons butter
6 tablespoons all-purpose flour
3 cups milk
2 cups shredded mild Cheddar cheese
¼ teaspoon dry mustard powder
salt to taste
⅛ teaspoon ground black pepper
1 cup crushed corn flake cereal
2 tablespoons butter, melted

DIRECTIONS:

Step 1
Preheat oven to 400 degrees F (200 degrees C).

Step 2
Cook asparagus in a large pot of lightly salted boiling water until tender, 5 to 8 minutes. Drain well and set aside.

Step 3
Scoop yolks out of hard-cooked eggs and transfer to a bowl; mash yolks with a fork.

Step 4
Mash deviled ham spread, cream, onion, 3/4 teaspoon dry mustard powder, Worcestershire sauce, and 1/2 teaspoon salt into the yolks until thoroughly combined.

Step 5
Fill cavities in egg halves with the yolk mixture; set deviled eggs aside.

Step 6
Melt 6 tablespoons of butter in a saucepan over medium heat, and whisk flour into butter until smooth and bubbling.

Step 7
Whisk in milk, a little at a time, until the sauce is smooth and thickened; reduce heat to low and simmer for 5 minutes.

Step 8
Whisk in Cheddar cheese, 1/4 teaspoon dry mustard powder, salt to taste, and black pepper; stir sauce until cheese is melted and incorporated.

Step 9
Spread asparagus into the bottom of a 9x13-inch baking dish.

Step 10
Arrange the deviled eggs on top of asparagus; pour the cheese sauce evenly over the deviled eggs.

Step 11
Mix crushed corn flakes with 2 tablespoons melted butter in a bowl; sprinkle over the casserole.

Step 12
Bake in the preheated oven until the sauce bubbles and the topping is browned, about 20 minutes.

NUTRITION FACTS:

652 calories; protein 32.2g; carbohydrates 33.1g; fat 44.9g; cholesterol 414.1mg;

SPICY SWEET PEPPER POPPERS

Prep:
30 mins
Cook:
30 mins
Total:
1 hr
Servings:
15
Yield:
30 poppers

INGREDIENTS:

15 miniature multi-colored sweet peppers, halved lengthwise, seeds removed
2 tablespoons olive oil
½ red onion, diced
3 cloves garlic, crushed
1 pound ground mild Italian sausage
5 button mushrooms, diced
½ cup tomato paste
½ cup tomato sauce
1 teaspoon crushed red pepper
½ teaspoon dried oregano
½ teaspoon dried rosemary
½ teaspoon freshly ground black pepper
⅛ teaspoon dried thyme

DIRECTIONS:

Step 1
Preheat oven to 400 degrees F (200 degrees C). Line a rimmed baking sheet with parchment paper.

Step 2
Heat oil in a large pan over medium heat. Add onions and cook until translucent, 3 to 5 minutes. Add garlic and cook 1 more minute. Add Italian sausage and mushrooms; cook until meat is browned, 4 to 6 minutes. Drain.

Step 3
Place drained sausage mixture in a large mixing bowl along with tomato paste, tomato sauce, crushed red peppers, oregano, rosemary, black pepper, and thyme. Mix until well combined.

Step 4
Fill each pepper half with mixture and place on prepared baking sheet.

Step 5
Bake in preheated oven until cooked through, about 30 minutes.

NUTRITION FACTS:

110 calories; protein 5.1g; carbohydrates 5.6g; fat 7.6g; cholesterol 11.9mg;

CHAPTER 2: LUNCH RECIPES

TURKEY VEGGIE MEATLOAF CUPS

Prep:
20 mins
Cook:
25 mins
Additional:
5 mins
Total:
50 mins
Servings:
10
Yield:
20 mini meatloaf cups

INGREDIENTS:

2 cups coarsely chopped zucchini
1 ½ cups coarsely chopped onions
1 red bell pepper, coarsely chopped
1 pound extra lean ground turkey
½ cup uncooked couscous
1 egg
2 tablespoons Worcestershire sauce
1 tablespoon Dijon mustard
½ cup barbecue sauce, or as needed

DIRECTIONS:

Step 1
Preheat oven to 400 degrees F (200 degrees C). Spray 20 muffin cups with cooking spray.

Step 2
Place zucchini, onions, and red bell pepper into a food processor, and pulse several times until finely chopped but not liquefied. Place the vegetables into a bowl, and mix in ground turkey, couscous, egg, Worcestershire sauce, and Dijon mustard until thoroughly combined. Fill each prepared muffin cup about 3/4 full. Top each cup with about 1 teaspoon of barbecue sauce.

Step 3
Bake in the preheated oven until juices run clear, about 25 minutes.
Internal temperature of a muffin measured by an instant-read meat thermometer should be at least 160 degrees F (70 degrees C).
Let stand 5 minutes before serving.

NUTRITION FACTS:

119 calories; protein 13.2g; carbohydrates 13.6g; fat 1g; cholesterol 46.7mg; sodium 244.4mg.

ONION AND MUSHROOM SCRAMBLED EGGS

Prep:
15 mins
Cook:
20 mins
Total:
35 mins
Servings:
2
Yield:
2 servings

INGREDIENTS:

1 ½ tablespoons extra-virgin olive oil
1 (8 ounce) package sliced fresh mushrooms
1 onion, sliced
1 clove garlic, minced
1 ½ tablespoons Italian seasoning
5 eggs
2 tablespoons garlic and herb cheese spread (such as Boursin®)
salt and ground black pepper to taste
⅓ cup shredded mozzarella cheese

DIRECTIONS:

Step 1
Heat olive oil in a skillet over medium heat; cook and stir mushrooms, onion, and garlic until onion is browned, about 15 minutes. Season with Italian seasoning.

Step 2
Beat eggs with garlic and herb cheese spread in a bowl. Mixture will be slightly chunky. Season with salt and black pepper.

Step 3
Pour eggs in skillet over mushroom mixture; cook and stir until eggs are nearly set, about 1 minute.
Fold mozzarella cheese into eggs until just melted, about 30 seconds

NUTRITION FACTS:

416 calories; protein 23.9g; carbohydrates 13.3g; fat 31.3g; cholesterol 438.8mg; sodium 369.1mg

CREAMY, LEMONY POTATO SALAD

Prep:
20 mins
Cook:
35 mins
Additional:
8 hrs
Total:
8 hrs 55 mins
Servings:
8
Yield:
8 servings

INGREDIENTS:

6 russet potatoes
4 eggs
½ cup coleslaw dressing (such as Kraft®)
½ cup creamy salad dressing (such as Miracle Whip®)
¼ cup snipped fresh chives
salt and ground black pepper to taste
1 pinch paprika, or more to taste

DIRECTIONS:

Step 1
Place potatoes into a large pot with enough salted water to just cover; bring to a boil, reduce heat to medium-low, and simmer, turning occasionally, until fork-tender, about 20 minutes. Drain potatoes and set aside to cool.

Step 2
Place eggs in a saucepan and cover with water. Bring to a boil, remove from heat, and let eggs cook in hot water for 15 minutes. Remove eggs from hot water and rinse with cold water until cool. Peel and chop eggs; put into a large glass dish.

Step 3
Peel cooled potatoes and chop; add to eggs in glass dish.

Step 4
Stir coleslaw dressing and creamy salad dressing together in a bowl until smooth; add chives and stir. Pour dressing over the potatoes and eggs; stir to coat. Season salad with salt and pepper; dust with paprika.

Step 5
Cover dish with plastic wrap and refrigerate overnight

NUTRITION FACTS:

260 calories; protein 6.4g; carbohydrates 33.7g; fat 11.2g;

SPICY SWEET POTATO AND COCONUT SOUP

Prep:
10 mins
Cook:
55 mins
Total:
1 hr 5 mins
Servings:
6
Yield:
6 servings

INGREDIENTS:

1 ½ pounds orange-fleshed sweet potatoes
1 tablespoon vegetable oil
1 onion, chopped
1 (2 inch) piece fresh ginger root, thinly sliced
1 tablespoon red curry paste
1 (15 ounce) can unsweetened coconut milk
3 cups vegetable broth
3 ½ tablespoons lemon juice
1 teaspoon sea salt
1 tablespoon toasted sesame oil
½ cup chopped fresh cilantro

DIRECTIONS:

Step 1
Preheat the oven to 400 degrees F (200 degrees C). Place the sweet potatoes directly on the rack and bake until tender enough to easily pierce with a fork, about 45 minutes. Remove from the oven and allow to cool.

Step 2
Heat the oil in a large saucepan or soup pot over medium heat. Add the onion and ginger; cook and stir until tender, about 5 minutes. Stir in the curry paste and heat for 1 minute, then whisk in the coconut milk and vegetable broth. Bring to a boil, then reduce heat to low and simmer for about 5 minutes.

Step 3
Remove the skins from the sweet potatoes and cut into bite size chunks.
Add to the soup and cook for 5 more minutes so they can soak up the flavor.
Stir in lemon juice and season with salt. Ladle into bowls and garnish with a drizzle of sesame oil and a little bit of cilantro.

NUTRITION FACTS:

306 calories; protein 4.1g; carbohydrates 30.6g; fat 20g;

POTATO-FREE PALEO GNOCCHI

Prep:
20 mins
Cook:
26 mins
Total:
46 mins
Servings:
4
Yield:
4 servings

INGREDIENTS:

Step 1
Place a steamer insert into a saucepan and fill with water to just below the bottom of the steamer. Bring water to a boil. Add kabocha squash, cover, and steam until soft, 10 to 15 minutes.

Step 2
Transfer steamed squash to a bowl; mash with a fork or potato masher. Mix in cassava flour, 1 pinch of salt, and nutmeg until a dough forms.

Step 3
Dust a flat work surface with cassava flour. Divide dough into pieces and roll into 1-inch thick logs. Cut into 1-inch gnocchi. Arrange gnocchi on a tray lined with parchment paper.

Step 4
Heat olive oil in a small skillet over medium heat. Cook sage leaves until crisp, 30 seconds to 1 minute. Press down with a fork to break leaves into small pieces. Stir in 1 tablespoon plus 1 teaspoon coconut milk and saffron. Simmer sauce until flavors combine, about 2 minutes. Remove from heat.

Step 5
Bring a large pot of water to a boil. Add 1 pinch of salt. Slide gnocchi gently into the water; cook until they float to the surface, 4 to 5 minutes. Scoop out with a wire strainer and transfer to serving plates.

Step 6
Cover gnocchi with 1 tablespoon of sauce. Drizzle some balsamic vinegar on top.

NUTRITION FACTS:

213 calories; protein 2.1g; carbohydrates 42.6g; fat 4.9g; sodium 90.3mg.

CUCUMBER WATERMELON SALAD

Prep:
15 mins
Additional:
20 mins
Total:
35 mins
Servings:
4
Yield:
4 servings

INGREDIENTS:

1 large cucumber, halved lengthwise and thinly sliced crosswise
2 medium tomatoes, diced
1 small onion, thinly sliced
2 cups cubed seedless watermelon
3 tablespoons red wine vinegar
2 tablespoons olive oil
1 teaspoon sea salt
1 teaspoon white sugar
½ teaspoon dried oregano
½ teaspoon dried basil
½ teaspoon ground thyme
½ teaspoon ground black pepper

DIRECTIONS:

Step 1
Combine cucumber, tomatoes, onion, and watermelon in a large bowl.

Step 2
Mix vinegar, olive oil, salt, sugar, oregano, basil, thyme, and pepper together in a separate, smaller bowl and pour over salad. Stir to coat well.

Step 3
Cover and refrigerate for 20 minutes. Serve chilled.

NUTRITION FACTS:

120 calories; protein 1.7g; carbohydrates 14.6g; fat 7.1g;

MUSHROOM, SCALLION, AND CHEESE OMELET

Prep:
10 mins
Cook:
9 mins
Total:
19 mins
Servings:
1
Yield:
1 omelet

INGREDIENTS:

2 eggs
1 tablespoon milk
salt and ground black pepper to taste
1 teaspoon coconut oil
2 mushrooms, chopped
1 green onions (green parts only), minced
1 tablespoon shredded Cheddar cheese, or to taste

DIRECTIONS:

Step 1
Beat eggs together with milk, salt, and pepper in a bowl.

Step 2
Heat oil in a skillet over medium heat. Add mushrooms; cook and stir until softened, about 5 minutes. Mix in green onions; cook until slightly softened, about 1 minute. Pour in the beaten eggs. Cook and stir until the edges harden, 2 to 3 minutes. Flip and sprinkle Cheddar cheese on top. Cook until egg is set and cheese is melted, 1 to 2 minutes. Fold omelet in half; top with more Cheddar cheese.

NUTRITION FACTS:

213 calories; protein 14.7g; carbohydrates 3.9g; fat 16g; cholesterol 336.1mg; sodium 333.7mg

PRETZEL TOPPED SWEET POTATOES

Prep:
20 mins
Cook:
25 mins
Total:
45 mins
Servings:
12
Yield:
12 servings

INGREDIENTS:

13 pretzel rods, crushed
1 cup chopped pecans
1 cup fresh cranberries
1 cup packed light brown sugar
1 cup melted butter, divided
1 (32 ounce) can sweet potatoes, drained
1 (5 ounce) can evaporated milk
½ cup white sugar
1 teaspoon vanilla extract

DIRECTIONS:

Step 1
Preheat oven to 350 degrees F (175 degrees C). Grease a 9x13-inch baking dish.

Step 2
Combine pretzels, pecans, cranberries, brown sugar, and 1/2 cup melted butter together in a bowl.

Step 3
Beat sweet potatoes together in a bowl until smooth; add evaporated milk, sugar, vanilla extract, and remaining 1/2 cup melted butter and mix until smooth. Spoon mixture into the prepared baking dish; sprinkle pretzel mixture over the top.

Step 4
Bake in the preheated oven until edges are bubbling, 25 to 30 minutes.

NUTRITION FACTS:

428 calories; protein 4.2g; carbohydrates 53.5g; fat 23.3g; cholesterol 44.1mg; sodium 386.5mg.

SAUTEED RICE WITH KALE

Prep:
15 mins
Cook:
20 mins
Total:
35 mins
Servings:
6
Yield:
6 servings

INGREDIENTS:

1 cup chopped kale
3 tablespoons olive oil
1 tablespoon butter
1 small onion, diced
1 stalk celery, diced
½ cup sliced fresh mushrooms
½ green bell pepper, diced
2 cloves garlic, minced
2 cups cooked white rice
1 teaspoon dry mustard
2 pinches cayenne pepper
salt and ground black pepper to taste

DIRECTIONS:

Step 1
Place a steamer insert into a saucepan and fill with water to just below the bottom of the steamer. Bring the water to a boil. Add the kale, cover, and steam until just tender, 7 to 10 minutes.

Step 2
Heat olive oil and butter in a large skillet over medium heat; cook and stir onion, celery, mushrooms, green bell pepper, and garlic in the oil and butter mixture until the onion is tender, about 5 minutes. Stir kale and rice into the mixture, breaking the rice into grains with your spoon as you stir; season with dry mustard, cayenne pepper, salt, and black pepper. Cook and stir until the rice is hot, about 5 minutes.

NUTRITION FACTS:

321 calories; protein 5.4g; carbohydrates 52.8g; fat 9.4g; cholesterol 5.1mg;

TENDER ONION BAKED CHICKEN

Prep:
5 mins
Cook:
40 mins
Total:
45 mins
Servings:
4
Yield:
4 servings

INGREDIENTS:

10 chicken breast tenderloins or strips
¼ cup margarine, melted
salt and pepper to taste
1 (1 ounce) envelope dry onion soup mix

DIRECTIONS:

Step 1
Preheat oven to 350 degrees F (175 degrees C).

Step 2
Place chicken in a 9x13 inch baking dish. Pour melted margarine over the chicken strips. Season with salt and pepper, and sprinkle with dry onion soup mix.

Step 3
Bake 40 minutes in the preheated oven, or until chicken is no longer pink and juices run clear.

NUTRITION FACTS:

270 calories; protein 32.3g; carbohydrates 4.5g; fat 13.1g; cholesterol 79.8mg;

MAYO FREE CABBAGE SALAD

Prep:
10 mins
Additional:
1 hr
Total:
1 hr 10 mins
Servings:
10
Yield:
10 servings

INGREDIENTS:

½ cup canola oil
¼ cup red wine vinegar
1 tablespoon soy sauce
6 tablespoons white sugar
1 (8 ounce) package shredded cabbage
3 green onions, thinly sliced
⅓ cup slivered almonds
⅓ cup sunflower seed kernels (Optional)

DIRECTIONS:

Step 1
Mix canola oil, red wine vinegar, soy sauce, and sugar in a large bowl, mixing until sugar has dissolved. Toss cabbage, green onions, almonds, and sunflower seed kernels into the dressing. Cover bowl and refrigerate at least 1 hour before serving; slaw tastes better when chilled overnight.

NUTRITION FACTS:

172 calories; protein 1.2g; carbohydrates 11.9g; fat 13.6g; cholesterol 1.8mg; sodium 96.5mg

SWEET AND TANGY APPLE PORK CHOPS

Prep:
10 mins
Cook:
10 mins
Additional:
10 mins
Total:
30 mins
Servings:
4
Yield:
4 servings

INGREDIENTS:

3 tablespoons brown sugar
2 tablespoons honey mustard
1 teaspoon mustard powder
½ teaspoon ground cumin
½ teaspoon cayenne pepper (Optional)
½ teaspoon garlic powder
1 pound pork chops
2 tablespoons butter
¾ cup apple cider

DIRECTIONS:

Step 1
Mix brown sugar, honey mustard, mustard powder, cumin, cayenne pepper, and garlic powder together in a small bowl; rub onto pork chops and let sit on a plate for flavors to dissolve into pork chops, about 10 minutes.

Step 2
Melt butter in a large skillet over medium heat; add apple cider. Arrange coated pork chops in the skillet; cook until pork chops are browned, 5 to 7 minutes per side. An instant-read thermometer inserted into the center should read at least 145 degrees F (63 degrees C).

NUTRITION FACTS:

265 calories; protein 15.1g; carbohydrates 20.4g; fat 14g; cholesterol 54.1mg;

CURRIED MUSTARD GREENS WITH KIDNEY BEANS

Prep:
15 mins
Cook:
15 mins
Total:
30 mins
Servings:
4
Yield:
4 servings

INGREDIENTS:

1 bunch mustard greens
1 tablespoon ghee (clarified butter)
2 medium shallots, chopped
1 tablespoon minced fresh ginger root
1 pinch red pepper flakes
1 (15 ounce) can kidney beans, drained and rinsed
1 (15 ounce) can tomato sauce
2 teaspoons curry powder
½ cup half and half

DIRECTIONS:

Step 1
Bring a large pot of lightly salted water to a boil. Place greens in the pot, cover, and cook 7 minutes, or just until tender. Drain, and rinse under cold water.

Step 2
Heat the ghee in a skillet over medium-high heat, and cook the shallots until lightly brown. Stir in ginger, and season with red pepper. Mix in greens, kidney beans, tomato sauce, and curry powder. Stir in the half and half, and continue cooking until heated through.

NUTRITION FACTS:

223 calories; protein 10.6g; carbohydrates 31.7g; fat 7.6g; cholesterol 19.4mg;

CREAMED BROCCOLI SOUP

Prep:
20 mins
Cook:
45 mins
Total:
1 hr 5 mins
Servings:
6
Yield:
6 servings

INGREDIENTS:

3 tablespoons butter
1 onion, chopped
4 large carrots, chopped
1 clove garlic, chopped
4 cups water
4 tablespoons chicken bouillon powder
1 pound fresh broccoli florets
2 cups half-and-half
3 tablespoons all-purpose flour
¼ cup ice water
1 tablespoon soy sauce
½ teaspoon ground black pepper
¼ cup chopped parsley

DIRECTIONS:

Step 1
Melt butter in a saucepan over medium heat; add chopped onions, carrots, and garlic, and cook for 5 minutes, stirring occasionally until softened.

Step 2
In a medium-sized cooking pot, add 4 cups water and chicken bouillon granules and bring to boil. Add precooked onion mixture to soup pot. Add broccoli florets, reserving a few pieces to be added near the end of cooking time. Reduce heat and simmer, covered, for 15 to 20 minutes or until broccoli is just tender.

Step 3
In a blender or food processor,
puree soup in batches and return to pot.
Stir in half and half cream
and remaining broccoli florets.

Step 4
In a cup, mix flour with 1/4 cup cold water to form a thin liquid.

Step 5
Bring soup to boil; add flour mixture slowly, stirring constantly to thicken soup as desired. Add soy sauce, black pepper, and stir well. Garnish with chopped parsley (or carrot curls) when serving. Serve soup hot or cold.

NUTRITION FACTS:

247 calories; protein 7.5g; carbohydrates 20.2g; fat 16.3g;

CHAPTER 3: DINNER RECIPES

SPICY SALMON AND VEGETABLE BOWL

Prep:
20 mins
Cook:
15 mins
Total:
35 mins
Servings:
4
Yield:
4 servings

INGREDIENTS:

2 tablespoons chili garlic sauce (sambal)
3 tablespoons soy sauce
2 tablespoons sesame oil
1 ½ tablespoons brown sugar
1 tablespoon rice wine vinegar
4 (6 ounce) salmon fillets, cut into 1-inch squares
1 red bell pepper, seeded and cut into 1-inch squares
1 cup snow peas
4 carrots, peeled and thinly sliced
4 cups cooked jasmine rice
Non Stick Aluminum Foil

DIRECTIONS:

Step 1
Preheat the broiler to low heat.

Step 2
Whisk together the chili garlic sauce, 2 tablespoons of soy sauce, 1 tablespoon of sesame oil, sugar and vinegar until combined.

Step 3
Add the cut up salmon to the bowl and mix until coated.

Step 4
Line a cookie sheet with Non-Stick Foil and evenly spread out the salmon and cook under the broiler for 8 to 10 minutes or until browned and cooked throughout.

Step 5
Pour the remaining 1 tablespoon of sesame oil into a large frying pan on high heat and add in the bell peppers, snow peas and carrot and stir-fry for 3 to 4 minutes. Finish the vegetables by adding the remaining 1 tablespoon of soy sauce.

Step 6
Divide the rice into 4 portions and serve the cooked salmon and vegetables evenly.

Step 7
Optional Servings: Serve with a hard boiled egg or a fried egg.

NUTRITION FACTS:

581 calories; protein 42.4g; carbohydrates 60.7g; fat 17.4g; cholesterol 74.7mg;

HOMEMADE VEGETABLE BEEF SOUP

Prep:
10 mins
Cook:
5 hrs 45 mins
Total:
5 hrs 55 mins
Servings:
10
Yield:
10 servings

INGREDIENTS:

1 ½ pounds beef stew meat, cut into 1/2-inch cubes
2 (14 ounce) cans beef broth
1 (15 ounce) can green beans, drained
1 (15.25 ounce) can whole kernel corn, drained
1 (14.5 ounce) can tomato sauce
1 (6 ounce) can tomato paste
1 (46 fluid ounce) bottle tomato-vegetable juice cocktail (such as V8®)
¼ teaspoon garlic powder, or to taste
¼ tablespoon onion powder, or to taste
salt and ground black pepper, to taste

DIRECTIONS:

Step 1
Mix beef broth and beef stew meat in a large pot over medium heat. Bring broth to a simmer, reduce heat to low, and cook beef at a simmer until tender, about 45 minutes.

Step 2
Stir corn, green beans, tomato sauce, and tomato paste with the beef. Pour tomato-vegetable juice cocktail into the pot; season with garlic powder, onion powder, salt, and pepper. Bring the mixture to a boil, reduce heat to low, and cook for 5 hours.

NUTRITION FACTS:

178 calories; protein 16.7g; carbohydrates 18.3g; fat 4.6g; cholesterol 35.9mg;

LEMONY SALMON WITH WATERCRESS SALAD

Prep:
35 mins
Cook:
15 mins
Additional:
15 mins
Total:
65 mins

INGREDIENTS:

SALMON:

1 tablespoon honey
1 tablespoon lemon juice
1 tablespoon chopped shallot
2 ½ teaspoons olive oil, divided
¼ teaspoon lemon zest
3 (6 ounce) fillets salmon

LEMON-PEPPER SAUCE:

½ cup creme fraiche
1 ½ teaspoons lemon juice
¼ teaspoon lemon zest
1 pinch salt and ground black pepper to taste

SALAD:

1 ½ cups watercress, chopped
¼ cup chopped fresh dill
¼ cup chopped fresh tarragon
2 teaspoons lemon juice
2 teaspoons olive oil
1 pinch salt and ground black pepper to taste
1 lemon, cut into wedges

DIRECTIONS:

Instructions Checklist
Step 1
Whisk honey, 1 tablespoon lemon juice, shallot, 1 1/2 teaspoon olive oil, and 1/4 teaspoon lemon zest together in a shallow baking dish. Add salmon fillets and turn to coat. Cover and refrigerate until flavors combine, 15 minutes to 1 hour.

Step 2
Whisk creme fraiche, 1 1/2 teaspoon lemon juice, 1/4 teaspoon lemon zest, salt, and pepper together in a small bowl to make lemon-pepper sauce.

Step 3
Toss watercress, dill, and tarragon with 2 teaspoons lemon juice and 2 teaspoons olive oil in a bowl to make salad. Season with salt and pepper.

Step 4
Set an oven rack in the top part of the oven and preheat to 400 degrees F (200 degrees C). Line a baking sheet with aluminum foil; brush with remaining 1 teaspoon olive oil.

Step 5
Transfer salmon fillets, with marinade, to the prepared baking sheet.

Step 6
Bake in the preheated oven until salmon is just opaque in the center, about 15 minutes.

Step 7
Serve salmon with some salad and sauce on top.
Serve remaining sauce on the side.
Garnish with lemon wedges.

NUTRITION FACTS:

477 calories; protein 38g; carbohydrates 13.1g; fat 32.1g;

CARROT, TOMATO, AND SPINACH QUINOA PILAF WITH GROUND TURKEY

Prep:
20 mins
Cook:
40 mins
Total:
60 mins
Servings:
5

INGREDIENTS:

2 teaspoons olive oil
1 cup quinoa
½ onion, chopped
2 cups water
2 tablespoons chicken-flavored vegetable bouillon
1 teaspoon ground black pepper
1 teaspoon ground thyme
1 carrot, chopped
1 tomato, chopped
1 cup baby spinach
2 tablespoons olive oil
1 pound ground turkey, or more to taste (Optional)

1 (14.5 ounce) can black beans, rinsed and drained

DIRECTIONS:

Step 1
Heat 2 teaspoons olive oil in a saucepan over medium heat; cook and stir onion in hot oil until translucent, about 5 minutes. Reduce heat to medium-low, stir quinoa with the onion, and cook, stirring constantly, until the quinoa is lightly toasted, about 2 minutes.

Step 2
Pour water into the saucepan; add bouillon granules, black pepper, and thyme. Bring the liquid to a boil, place a cover on the saucepan, reduce heat to low, and cook at a simmer until the quinoa softens, about 5 minutes.

Step 3
Stir carrot into the quinoa mixture, replace cover, and continue to cook at a simmer until water is completely absorbed, about 10 minutes more.

Step 4
Remove saucepan from heat. Stir tomato and baby spinach into the quinoa mixture until the spinach wilts, about 2 minutes.

Step 5
Heat 2 tablespoons olive oil in large skillet over medium-high heat. Cook and stir turkey in the hot skillet until browned and crumbly, 5 to 7 minutes; drain and discard grease. Reduce heat to medium-low. Stir black beans with the turkey; cook and stir until the beans are hot, 2 to 3 minutes; add the quinoa mixture, stir, and cook until heated through, about 5 minutes more.

NUTRITION FACTS:

422 calories; protein 28.6g; carbohydrates 40.8g; fat 16.6g; cholesterol 66.9mg; sodium 396mg.

SAVORY VEGETABLE BEEF STEW

Prep:
30 mins
Cook:
2 hrs 30 mins
Total:
2 hrs 60 mins

INGREDIENTS:

3 pounds beef stew meat, cut into 1-inch pieces
⅓ cup Italian salad dressing
2 cups water
2 teaspoons beef bouillon granules
1 (14.5 ounce) can diced tomatoes, undrained
1 (10.5 ounce) can condensed beef broth
1 (8 ounce) can tomato sauce
1 clove garlic, minced
1 bay leaf
1 teaspoon salt
1 teaspoon dried oregano
½ teaspoon ground black pepper
6 small potatoes, quartered
6 carrots, cut into 1-inch pieces
1 green bell pepper, cut into 1/2-inch dice
1 onion, chopped
3 tablespoons all-purpose flour
3 tablespoons cold water

DIRECTIONS:

Step 1
Heat a large skillet or Dutch oven over medium heat; cook and stir beef stew meat and Italian dressing until meat is evenly browned, about 5 minutes. Add 2 cups water, beef bouillon, diced tomatoes, beef broth, tomato sauce, garlic, bay leaf, salt, oregano, and pepper to skillet; bring to a boil. Reduce heat to medium-low, cover, and simmer until meat is tender, about 1 1/2 hours.

Step 2
Place potatoes, carrots, bell pepper, and onion in stew; cover and simmer over medium-low heat until vegetables are tender, about 45 minutes.

Step 3
Combine flour and cold water in a small bowl; mix until smooth. Stir flour mixture into stew, bring to a boil; cook and stir until stew is thickened, about 2 minutes. Discard bay leaf before serving.

NUTRITION FACTS:

342 calories; protein 21.8g; carbohydrates 23.7g; fat 17.5g; cholesterol 62.7mg;

AMAZING GRILLED CHICKEN AND PINEAPPLE

Prep:
15 mins
Cook:
15 mins
Additional:
1 day
Total:
1 day
Servings:
4
Yield:
4 chicken breasts

INGREDIENTS:

CHICKEN:

1 (13.5 ounce) can light coconut milk
1 ½ cups Hawaiian marinade
2 tablespoons garlic powder
4 skinless, boneless chicken breast halves

PINEAPPLE:

1 (13.5 ounce) can light coconut milk
2 tablespoons ground cinnamon
1 tablespoon vanilla extract
1 tablespoon butter flavoring
8 slices fresh pineapple, or more to taste

DIRECTIONS:

Step 1
Combine coconut milk, Hawaiian marinade, and garlic powder in a dish large enough to marinate the chicken breasts. Add chicken. Cover and marinate in the refrigerator, turning every 3 to 4 hours, about 24 hours.

Step 2
Combine coconut milk, cinnamon, vanilla extract, and butter flavoring in a dish. Add pineapple. Cover and marinate in the refrigerator, at least 1 hour.

Step 3
Preheat an outdoor grill for high heat and lightly oil the grate. Place chicken on hot grill; discard marinade. Cook chicken, without pressing or poking, and flipping only twice, until no longer pink in the center and the juices run clear, 5 to 7 minutes per side. An instant-read thermometer inserted into the center should read at least 165 degrees F (74 degrees C). Transfer chicken to a platter; let rest for 4 to 5 minutes.

Step 4

Place pineapple on the hot grill and cook on medium-high heat for 2 to 3 minutes per side. Transfer grilled pineapple to the platter with the chicken.

NUTRITION FACTS:

587 calories; protein 34.3g; carbohydrates 63.6g; fat 20.2g; cholesterol 67.2mg;

FRESH VEGETABLE STIR-FRY WITH PEPPERY ORANGE BEEF

Prep:
15 mins
Cook:
45 mins
Total:
60 mins
Servings:
8
Yield:
8 servings

INGREDIENTS:

2 cups uncooked long grain white rice
1 quart water
1 tablespoon light sesame oil
4 cloves garlic, crushed
5 tablespoons butter
2 pounds flank steak, cut into thin strips
salt to taste
4 teaspoons red pepper flakes
3 ½ tablespoons teriyaki sauce
12 ounces fresh mushrooms, sliced

1 large sweet onion, sliced
½ head cabbage, sliced into strips
1 green bell pepper, cut into strips
1 red bell pepper, cut into strips
1 yellow bell pepper, cut into strips
1 teaspoon cornstarch
1 tablespoon brown sugar
½ cup beef broth
2 tablespoons orange jam
1 (5 ounce) can chow mein noodles
mustard powder to taste

DIRECTIONS:

Step 1
In a pot, bring the rice and water to a boil. Cover, reduce heat to low, and simmer 20 minutes.

Step 2
Heat the sesame oil in a skillet over medium heat, and cook 2 cloves garlic for 2 minutes, until tender. Melt the butter in the skillet. Season the beef with salt and 2 teaspoons red pepper flakes. Cook and stir the beef in the skillet 10 minutes, until evenly brown. Reserving pan drippings, transfer the cooked beef to a bowl, and coat with 3 tablespoons teriyaki sauce.

Step 3
Melt the remaining butter in a separate skillet over medium heat, and cook the remaining garlic 2 minutes, until tender. Remove garlic, and set aside. Stir the mushrooms and onions into the skillet, and cook until onions are tender. Mix in the cabbage, green bell pepper, red bell pepper, and yellow bell pepper. Cook 3 minutes, until tender but

still crisp. Remove skillet from heat, and mix in remaining 1/2 tablespoon teriyaki sauce and 1/2 the reserved pan drippings.

Step 4
Heat the remaining pan drippings in the skillet over medium heat. Mix in the remaining red pepper flakes, teriyaki sauce from the beef bowl, the reserved garlic, cornstarch, brown sugar, beef broth, and orange jam. Cook 5 minutes, until thickened. Remove garlic, and stir in the beef to coat.

Step 5
Serve the beef and vegetables, along with some of the skillet juices, over the cooked rice. Top with chow mein noodles, and sprinkle with mustard powder.

NUTRITION FACTS:

566 calories; protein 24.2g; carbohydrates 67.8g; fat 22.3g; cholesterol 54.8mg;

BACON ROSEMARY STUFFED MUSHROOMS

Prep:
20 mins
Cook:
25 mins
Total:
45 mins
Servings:
6
Yield:
6 servings

INGREDIENTS:

2 tablespoons butter
1 onion, chopped
1 (8 ounce) package mushrooms, stems removed and chopped and caps reserved
4 slices bacon, chopped
1 ¼ cups shredded Edam cheese
2 sprigs fresh rosemary, chopped

DIRECTIONS:

Step 1
Preheat oven to 400 degrees F (200 degrees C).

Step 2
Melt butter in a skillet over medium heat and cook onion until soft and translucent, about 5 minutes. Add chopped mushroom stems and cook until soft, 5 to 7 minutes.

Step 3
Place bacon in a large skillet and cook over medium-high heat until evenly browned, about 10 minutes.
Drain bacon pieces on paper towels and add
to mushroom mixture.
Stir in Edam cheese and rosemary
and mix to combine.
Fill mushroom caps with mixture
and place on a baking sheet.

Step 4
Bake in the preheated oven until filling is lightly browned and cheese is melted, 15 to 20 minutes.

NUTRITION FACTS:

174 calories; protein 9.7g; carbohydrates 5.2g; fat 13.1g; cholesterol 37.8mg; sodium 397.3mg.

CLASSIC BEEF STUFFED PEPPERS

Prep:
20 mins
Cook:
1 hr
Total:
1 hr 20 mins
Servings:
6
Yield:
6 servings

INGREDIENTS:

6 red bell peppers - tops and seeds removed
3 eggs, beaten
3 cups meatless spaghetti sauce
1 ¼ cups instant rice
¼ cup finely chopped onion
1 teaspoon salt
1 ½ teaspoons Worcestershire sauce
1 pinch ground black pepper
1 ½ pounds lean ground beef
2 cups meatless spaghetti sauce
6 tablespoons shredded Cheddar cheese, divided

DIRECTIONS:

Step 1
Preheat oven to 350 degrees F (175 degrees C).

Step 2
Bring a large saucepan of water to a boil, reduce heat to medium, and cook red bell peppers in the boiling water until slightly softened, about 5 minutes. Drain and rinse peppers with cold water.

Step 3
Stir eggs, 3 cups of spaghetti sauce, instant rice, onion, salt, Worcestershire sauce, and black pepper together in a bowl. Crumble ground beef into the mixture and stir until ground beef is thoroughly combined with sauce and rice mixture.

Step 4
Stand peppers in a large baking dish and fill each pepper with beef mixture. Pour 2 cups spaghetti sauce over the peppers. Cover dish with aluminum foil.

Step 5
Bake in the preheated oven until peppers are tender, the filling is set, and an instant-read meat thermometer inserted into the middle of a pepper reads at least 160 degrees F (70 degrees C), 55 to 60 minutes. Uncover and top each pepper with 1 tablespoon Cheddar cheese.

NUTRITION FACTS:

595 calories; protein 34.9g; carbohydrates 53.4g; fat 25.7g; cholesterol 183.3mg;

CRANBERRY AND TURKEY SALAD

Prep:
10 mins
Total:
10 mins
Servings:
4
Yield:
4 servings

INGREDIENTS:

3 cups chopped cooked turkey
½ cup dried cranberries
½ cup sliced almonds
2 stalks celery, chopped
2 tablespoons mayonnaise

DIRECTIONS:

Step 1
Mix turkey, cranberries, almonds, celery, and mayonnaise in a bowl until well blended.

NUTRITION FACTS:

347 calories; protein 33.4g; carbohydrates 15.4g; fat 16.7g; cholesterol 82.4mg; sodium 128.7mg.

TURKEY VEGETABLE SOUP

Prep:
30 mins
Cook:
1 hr 30 mins
Total:
1 hr 60 mins
Servings:
10
Yield:
10 servings

INGREDIENTS:

6 cups turkey pan drippings, fat skimmed
8 cups water
2 turkey legs
2 cloves garlic, crushed
1 bay leaf
½ teaspoon dried thyme
ground black pepper to taste
¼ cup all-purpose flour
½ cup milk
2 cups cubed cooked turkey
6 red potatoes, diced
½ onion, quartered and sliced
3 carrots, sliced
2 stalks celery, sliced

DIRECTIONS:

Step 1
In a large stock pot, stir together the turkey drippings, water, turkey legs, garlic, bay leaf, thyme, and black pepper. Bring to a boil, reduce heat to a simmer, and cover the pot; simmer until the turkey meat is starting to fall from the bones, about 30 minutes. Remove turkey legs, and pick the meat from the bones; return the leg meat to the soup.

Step 2
Whisk 1/4 cup of flour with 1/2 cup of milk in a bowl until smooth, and stir the mixture into the soup. Return soup to simmer, stirring constantly, and cook until thickened, about 30 more minutes. Mix in the cubed cooked turkey meat, red potatoes, onion, carrots, and celery; cover the pot again, and simmer until the celery is tender, about 30 more minutes.

NUTRITION FACTS:

194 calories; protein 25g; carbohydrates 11g; fat 4.9g; cholesterol 61.4mg;

PEANUT BUTTER SAUCE CHICKEN

Prep:
10 mins
Cook:
15 mins
Total:
25 mins
Servings:
4
Yield:
4 servings

INGREDIENTS:

1 tablespoon sesame oil
½ teaspoon minced garlic
1 pinch salt
¼ cup pine nuts
2 cooked, boneless chicken breast halves, diced
1 tablespoon peanut butter
1 dash soy sauce
3 pickled jalapeno pepper slices, chopped
½ cup water

DIRECTIONS:

Step 1
Heat the sesame oil in a skillet over medium heat. Stir in the garlic and salt. Cook and stir 1 minute, then stir in the pine nuts, and cook until golden, about 5 minutes. Add the diced chicken breast, and cook a few minutes to reheat. Stir in the peanut butter, soy sauce, and jalapeno pepper until the peanut butter has melted. Pour in the water, and bring to a simmer. Cook and stir until the sauce has thickened, about 5 minutes more.

NUTRITION FACTS:

171 calories; protein 13.2g; carbohydrates 2.3g; fat 12.5g; cholesterol 27.6mg; sodium 69.6mg.

ASIAGO TOASTED CHEESE PUFFS

Prep:
10 mins
Cook:
3 mins
Total:
13 mins
Servings:
12
Yield:
12 servings

INGREDIENTS:

1 cup grated Asiago cheese
1 teaspoon pressed garlic
⅓ cup mayonnaise
1 teaspoon dried oregano
1 teaspoon dried thyme
1 teaspoon dried parsley
1 pinch salt
1 pinch ground black pepper
1 French baguette, thinly sliced

DIRECTIONS:

Step 1
Preheat the broiler.

Step 2
In a mixing bowl, combine the Asiago, garlic, mayonnaise, oregano, thyme, parsley, salt and pepper. If the mixture does not hold together well, add more mayonnaise, if desired.

Step 3
On a baking sheet, arrange the baguette slices in a single layer. Spread the Asiago mixture on the slices. Broil for 3 minutes, or until the cheese is melted and lightly browned. Serve immediately.

NUTRITION FACTS:

187 calories; protein 6.8g; carbohydrates 21.9g; fat 8.1g; cholesterol 10.4mg;

SPICY ORANGE CHICKEN

Prep:
20 mins
Cook:
25 mins
Additional:
1 hr
Total:
1 hr 45 mins
Servings:
6
Yield:
6 servings

INGREDIENTS:

1 cup orange juice
⅓ cup brown sugar
⅓ cup rice vinegar
2 tablespoons fish sauce
1 tablespoon soy sauce
1 tablespoon fresh ginger root, grated
1 teaspoon crushed red pepper flakes
2 pounds skinless, boneless chicken thighs, cut into chunks
1 bunch green onions, sliced, white parts and tops separated
1 fresh jalapeno pepper, sliced into rings
1 red bell pepper, cut into 2 inch pieces
½ cup sugar snap peas
4 cloves garlic, minced

2 tablespoons grated orange zest
1 bunch cilantro leaves, for garnish

DIRECTIONS:

Step 1
Whisk orange juice, brown sugar, rice vinegar, fish sauce, soy sauce, ginger, and crushed red pepper flakes in a large bowl.

Step 2
Mix in chicken pieces and toss to evenly coat. Cover the bowl with plastic wrap and marinate in the refrigerator for 1 hour.

Step 3
Remove chicken from refrigerator and drain thoroughly in colander, reserving marinade.

Step 4
Heat a large non-stick skillet over high heat. Cook and stir chicken for 2 minutes; spoon out any excess liquid.

Step 5
Continue to cook and stir until chicken caramelizes, 6 to 7 minutes.

Step 6
Stir in white portions of green onions, garlic, and orange zest; cook and stir 2 to 3 minutes.

Step 7
Pour in half of reserved marinade. Simmer until reduced and thickened, 3 to 4 minutes.

Step 8

Stir in jalapeno pepper, bell pepper, and sugar snap peas; cook and stir until vegetables are warmed, about 2 minutes.

Step 9
Stir in green portions of green onions; cook and stir 1 minute.

Step 10
Remove from heat. Garnish with cilantro and serve.

NUTRITION FACTS:

325 calories; protein 31g; carbohydrates 25.2g; fat 10.8g; cholesterol 103.4mg; sodium 627mg.

CHAPTER 4: SMOOTHIE RECIPES

BANANA-DATE SHAKE

Prep:
5 mins
Total:
5 mins
Servings:
1
Yield:
1 cup

INGREDIENTS:

¾ cup plain soy milk
1 frozen banana, halved
2 large dates, pitted and chopped
½ tablespoon ground cinnamon, or to taste

DIRECTIONS:

Step 1
Combine soy milk, banana, dates, and cinnamon in a blender. Blend until smooth. Serve.

NUTRITION FACTS:

372 calories; protein 8.8g; carbohydrates 83.7g; fat 3.8g; sodium 95.6mg.

SWEET POTATO-BANANA SMOOTHIE

Prep:
10 mins
Total:
10 mins
Servings:
1
Yield:
1 serving

INGREDIENTS:

1 small banana
½ small cooked sweet potato
½ cup cottage cheese
½ cup low-fat milk
5 cubes ice, or as needed
1 tablespoon cocoa powder
1 tablespoon molasses
1 tablespoon honey
⅛ teaspoon almond extract

DIRECTIONS:

Step 1
Blend banana, sweet potato, cottage cheese, milk, ice, cocoa powder, molasses, honey, and almond extract together in a high-power blender until smooth.

NUTRITION FACTS:

455 calories; protein 21.4g; carbohydrates 78.8g; fat 8.7g; cholesterol 26.6mg; sodium 659.4mg

STRAWBERRY-ORANGE CREME SMOOTHIES

Prep:
5 mins
Total:
5 mins
Servings:
2
Yield:
2 servings

INGREDIENTS:

2 (5.3 ounce) containers Greek 100 Orange Creme yogurt
1 cup fresh strawberries, hulled
½ cup ice cubes (Optional)
¼ cup orange juice

DIRECTIONS:

Step 1
In blender, place ingredients. Cover; blend on high speed about 10 seconds or until smooth.

Step 2
Pour into 2 glasses. Serve immediately.

NUTRITION FACTS:

137 calories; protein 12.7g; carbohydrates 20.8g; fat 0.3g; cholesterol 0.1mg; sodium 103.1mg.

VANILLA BANAMANGO SMOOTHIE

Prep:
15 mins
Total:
15 mins
Servings:
2
Yield:
2 servings

INGREDIENTS:

¼ cup orange juice, or to taste
1 mango, sliced
1 frozen banana, sliced
2 baby carrots
1 (6 ounce) container vanilla yogurt
2 ice cubes, or as desired
1 teaspoon ground ginger

DIRECTIONS:

Step 1
Pour orange juice into the pitcher of a blender and add mango, frozen banana, carrots, vanilla yogurt, ice cubes, and ginger. Pulse several times to crush ice, then blend until smooth, 30 seconds to 1 minute.

NUTRITION FACTS:

191 calories; protein 5.5g; carbohydrates 41.8g; fat 1.6g; cholesterol 4.3mg; sodium 59.4mg.

ZUCCHINI SMOOTHIE

Prep:
5 mins
Total:
5 mins
Servings:
1
Yield:
1 serving

INGREDIENTS:

½ cup ice cubes, or as needed (Optional)
½ zucchini, shredded
½ frozen banana
½ cup orange juice

DIRECTIONS:

Step 1
Combine ice cubes, zucchini, banana, and orange juice in a blender. Blend until smooth.

NUTRITION FACTS:

118 calories; protein 2.2g; carbohydrates 28.3g; fat 0.5g; sodium 11.4mg.

www.ingramcontent.com/pod-product-compliance
Lightning Source LLC
Chambersburg PA
CBHW070934080526
44589CB00013B/1513